Fitness Motivation and Goal Setting

Unlocking Your Potential for Lifelong Health and Wellness.

Eric Uroh

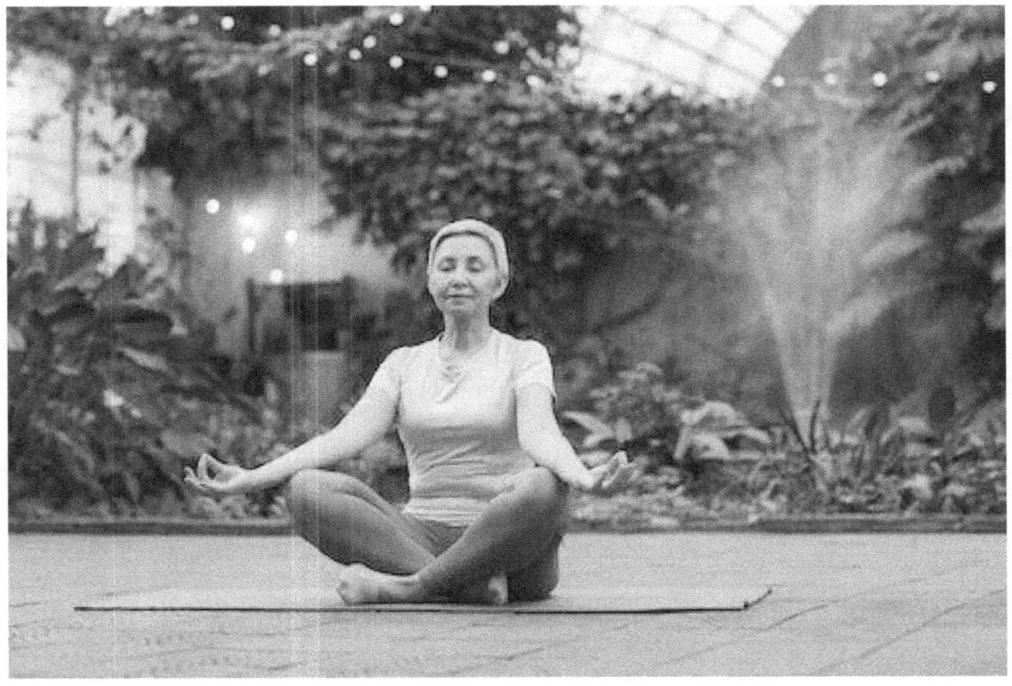

TABLE OF CONTENTS

Introduction

Welcome, and a brief overview of the book's purpose.
The importance of motivation and goal setting in fitness.
Setting the stage for the reader's fitness journey.

Chapter 1: Understanding Your Why

The power of intrinsic motivation.
Identifying and defining personal fitness goals.
Connecting fitness goals to personal values and desires.
Exercises and reflection prompts to help readers discover their "why."

Chapter 2: Goal Setting Techniques

The SMART goal framework (Specific, Measurable, Achievable, Relevant, Time-bound).
Long-term vs. short-term goals.
Breaking down big goals into manageable milestones.
Setting process-oriented goals.

Chapter 3: Crafting Your Fitness Plan

Choosing the right type of exercise (e.g., cardio, strength training, flexibility).
Customizing a workout plan based on individual fitness goals.
Creating a balanced and sustainable workout routine.
Incorporating variety to prevent boredom and plateaus.

Chapter 4: Nutrition and Diet for Success

The role of nutrition in fitness and goal attainment.
Establishing healthy eating habits.
Tailoring dietary choices to fitness objectives.

Meal planning and tracking food intake.

Chapter 5: Overcoming Obstacles

Common obstacles to motivation and goal achievement.
Strategies for overcoming setbacks and challenges.
Dealing with plateaus and moments of self-doubt.
Building resilience and mental toughness.

Chapter 6: Staying Motivated

Motivational techniques and strategies.
The power of visualization and positive self-talk.
Accountability partners and support systems.
Monitoring progress and celebrating victories.

Chapter 7: Maintaining Momentum

Strategies for long-term commitment to fitness.
Adjusting goals as circumstances change.
Avoiding burnout and finding balance in life.
The role of rest and recovery in maintaining motivation.

Chapter 8: Case Studies and Success Stories

Real-life examples of individuals who achieved their fitness goals.
Their journeys, challenges, and the strategies they used.
Inspiration for readers to see what's possible.

Chapter 9: Resources and Tools

Recommended apps, websites, and fitness tracking tools.
Books, podcasts, and online communities for continued motivation.
Creating a personal fitness toolkit.

Conclusion

Summing up key takeaways from the book.
Encouragement and motivation for readers to start their fitness journey.
Reminding readers that fitness is a lifelong pursuit.
Introduction: Fitness Motivation and Goal Setting

In a world filled with countless distractions and demands, embarking on a journey to achieve your fitness goals can be a daunting task. It's a path often marked by uncertainty, self-doubt, and the ever-present temptation to give in to momentary comfort. Yet, within the realm of fitness, as in many aspects of life, two guiding lights shine brighter than all the rest: motivation and goal setting.

Welcome to "Fitness Motivation and Goal Setting," an eBook designed to empower you on your transformative journey toward a healthier, more vibrant you. Within these pages, you'll discover the twin pillars that can make the seemingly impossible not only possible but also deeply rewarding.

1. The Importance of Motivation and Goal Setting in Fitness

Imagine having an unshakable source of motivation that propels you out of bed each morning, eager to conquer your workouts and make healthy choices throughout the day. Picture a roadmap to your ideal self, complete with signposts marking each achievement along the way. This is the power of motivation and goal-setting in fitness.

Motivation is the spark that ignites your inner fire, propelling you forward even when the going gets tough. It's the driving force that transforms "I should exercise" into "I can't wait to exercise." Goal setting, on the other hand, provides the structure and direction necessary to turn dreams into concrete, achievable realities. By defining your objectives, you create a roadmap for success and a sense of purpose that guides your every step.

2. Setting the Stage for Your Fitness Journey

Before we dive into the practical techniques and strategies that will shape your path to fitness, it's important to acknowledge that every fitness journey is unique. Your starting point, your aspirations, and your motivations are entirely your own. The journey begins with understanding where you are now and where you want to go.

In this eBook, we'll explore various facets of your fitness journey, including:

Chapter 1: Understanding Your Why – We'll delve into the power of intrinsic motivation, helping you identify and define your personal fitness goals and connect them to your deepest values and desires.

Chapter 2: Goal Setting Techniques – You'll learn how to set SMART goals, distinguish between long-term and short-term objectives, and break down daunting aspirations into manageable milestones.

Chapter 3: Crafting Your Fitness Plan – Discover how to choose the right type of exercise, customize a workout plan tailored to your goals, and maintain variety to prevent boredom and plateaus.

Chapter 4: Nutrition and Diet for Success – Explore the role of nutrition in achieving your goals, developing healthy eating habits, and learning how to plan and track your food intake effectively.

Chapter 5: Overcoming Obstacles – Navigate common challenges on your journey, develop strategies to overcome setbacks and doubts, and build the resilience needed to persevere.

Chapter 6: Staying Motivated – Dive into motivational techniques, the power of visualization, and the importance of accountability and support systems.

Chapter 7: Maintaining Momentum – Learn how to sustain your commitment to fitness, adjust goals as life evolves, and find a balance to avoid burnout.

Chapter 8: Case Studies and Success Stories – Draw inspiration from real-life examples of individuals who achieved their fitness goals, discovering the strategies that worked for them.

Chapter 9: Resources and Tools – Explore recommended apps, websites, and fitness-tracking tools, along with books, podcasts, and communities to keep you motivated.

Conclusion – We'll wrap up by summarizing key takeaways and offering encouragement to embark on your lifelong fitness journey.

With "Fitness Motivation and Goal Setting" as your guide, you'll gain the knowledge and tools needed to set forth on a transformative path, one that will not only enhance your physical well-being but also empower you to unlock your full potential in every aspect of your life. So, let's embark on this journey together, and remember: fitness is not just a destination; it's a lifelong pursuit of your best self.

Chapter 1: Understanding Your Why

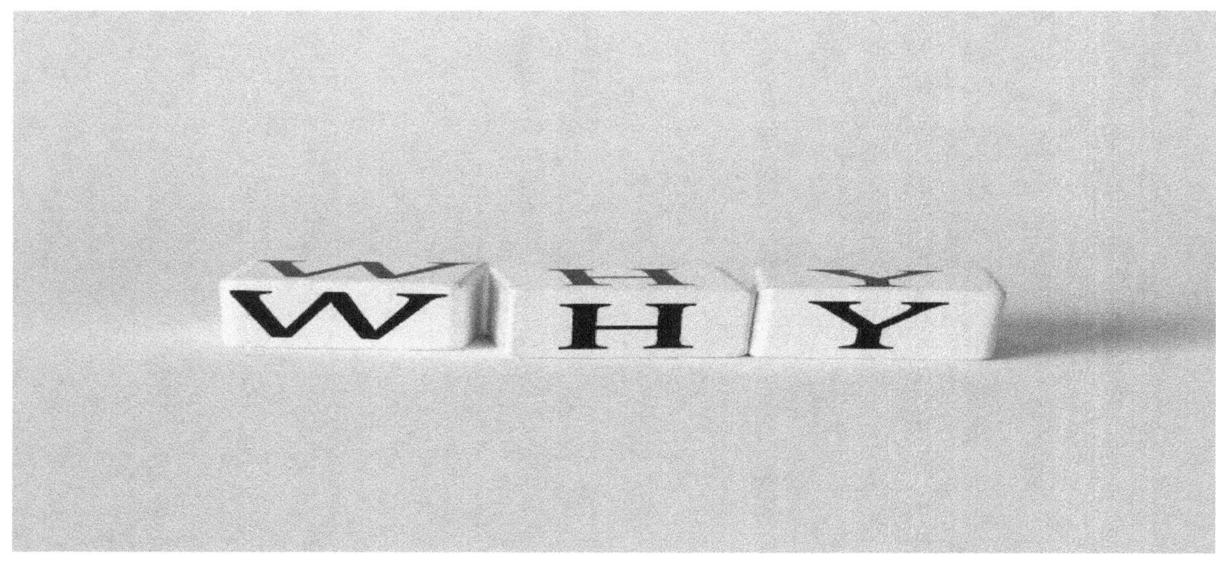

The Power of Intrinsic Motivation

Motivation is the heartbeat of any successful fitness journey. It's the driving force that propels you out of bed for that early morning jog or inspires you to make wholesome food choices when tempted by indulgence. While there are many sources of motivation, intrinsic motivation stands as a powerful beacon that can illuminate your path toward lasting fitness success.

Intrinsic motivation is the kind that comes from within. It's not motivated by external factors like praise or rewards; instead, it's deeply rooted in your own desires, values, and aspirations. It's the force that compels you to pursue fitness not because you feel you should, but because you genuinely want to.

Helping You Identify and Define Your Personal Fitness Goals

To harness the power of intrinsic motivation, you must first identify and define your personal fitness goals. These goals are your unique vision for what you want to achieve through fitness, and they're as diverse as the individuals embarking on this journey.

Begin by reflecting on what fitness means to you. Is it about losing weight, gaining muscle, improving endurance, or simply feeling more energetic and vital in your daily life? Your goals should resonate with your innermost desires and aspirations, not someone else's expectations or societal pressures.

As you ponder your fitness objectives, remember that they can encompass a wide spectrum, from short-term to long-term and from specific to holistic. The key is to create a set of goals that are meaningful to you, ones that will fuel your motivation even on the toughest of days.

Connect Them to Your Deepest Values and Desires

Now, let's delve deeper. Your fitness goals aren't isolated entities; they are intrinsically connected to your deepest values and desires. These values represent what matters most to you in life, and your fitness journey can become a profound expression of those values.

For example, if you value health and longevity, your fitness goals might include activities that promote overall well-being, such as regular exercise and a balanced diet. If you value personal growth and self-discovery, your goals might involve challenging yourself to reach new levels of fitness competence.

To connect your fitness goals to your values, ask yourself why achieving these goals is important to you. What will you gain by attaining them? How will they align with your values and bring you closer to living the life you desire?

Imagine, for a moment, a future where you've achieved your fitness goals. Visualize how it aligns with your values and contributes to your overall happiness and fulfillment. This exercise not only strengthens your commitment but also adds depth and meaning to your fitness journey.

By understanding your why—tapping into the wellspring of intrinsic motivation—you're setting a solid foundation for the exciting and transformative path that lies ahead. In the chapters to come, we'll explore techniques and strategies to transform your intrinsic motivation into concrete action and results. Your journey to fitness success begins with clarity, purpose, and the unwavering commitment to your unique why.

Chapter 2: Goal Setting Techniques

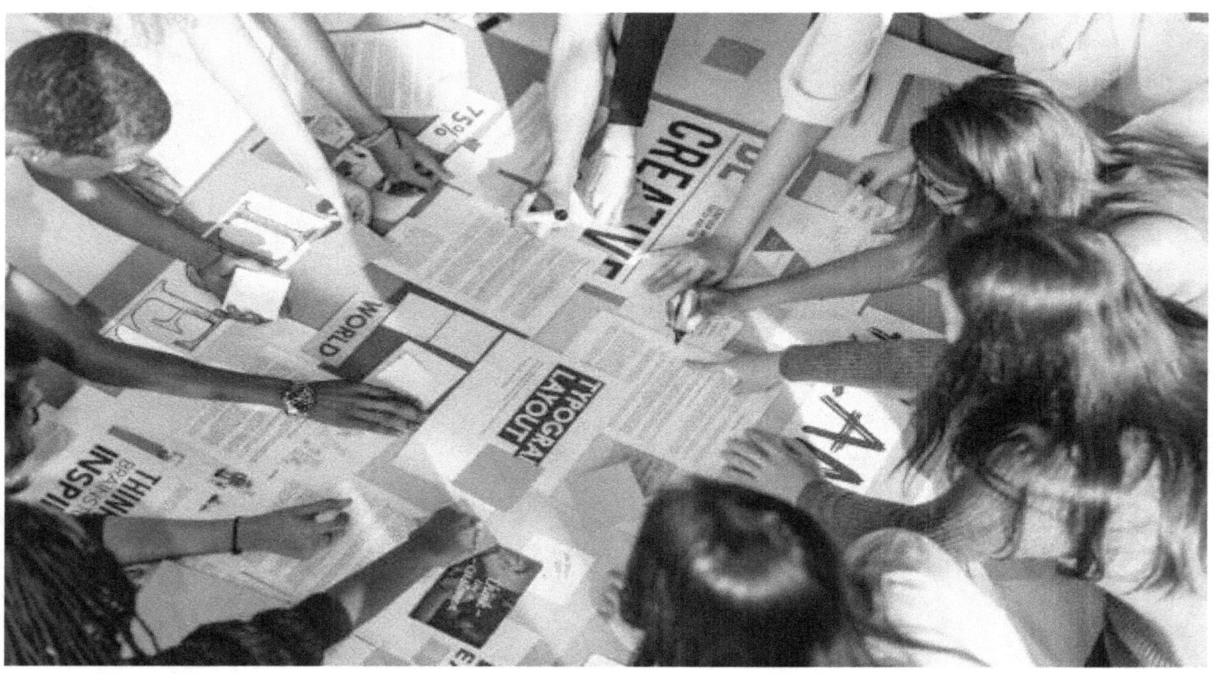

Set SMART Goals

As you embark on your journey to fitness, setting clear and well-defined goals is your compass, steering you in the direction of success. One of the most effective techniques for crafting goals that lead to meaningful progress is using the SMART criteria: Specific, Measurable, Achievable, Relevant, and Time-bound.

Specific: Your fitness goals should be crystal clear and focused. Instead of a vague goal like "get fit," aim for something like "run a 5k race in six months." The more specific your goal, the easier it is to visualize and work towards.

Measurable: Goals should be quantifiable so that you can track your progress. Rather than saying "lose weight," specify "lose 15 pounds" or "reduce body fat percentage by 5%."

Achievable: While ambition is essential, your goals should also be realistic. Set yourself up for success by ensuring that your goals are within reach. Consider your current fitness level, time constraints, and available resources.

Relevant: Your fitness goals should align with your larger aspirations and values. Ask yourself if your goal is genuinely relevant to your life and if it contributes to your overall well-being.

Time-bound: Every goal needs a deadline. Establishing a timeframe creates a sense of urgency and helps you stay accountable. For example, set a goal to "run a 5k race in six months" rather than just "someday."

Distinguish Between Long-Term and Short-Term Objectives

Goals can be categorized as either long-term or short-term, each serving a unique purpose in your fitness journey.

Long-term goals are your destination, the ultimate achievements you aim to realize over an extended period. They might encompass year-long objectives like "lose 50 pounds" or "complete a marathon." Long-term goals provide a sense of purpose and direction.

Short-term goals are the stepping stones that guide you toward your long-term aspirations. These goals are often smaller and more achievable in the near future. For instance, if your long-term goal is to lose 50 pounds, your short-term goals could involve weekly or monthly targets for weight loss. Short-term goals offer a sense of accomplishment and help maintain your motivation as you progress.

Break Down Daunting Aspirations into Manageable Milestones

It's common to feel overwhelmed when faced with significant fitness aspirations. Whether you're aiming to transform your body, build endurance, or master a new skill, breaking down daunting goals into manageable milestones is a game-changer.

Consider this: if your long-term goal is to complete a marathon, the thought of running 26.2 miles can be intimidating. However, by dividing it into smaller milestones, like running a 5k, then a half marathon, and gradually increasing your distance, you'll find that the journey becomes far less intimidating.

Breaking down your goals into smaller steps not only makes them more achievable but also provides a sense of progress and accomplishment along the way. Each milestone you reach serves as motivation to keep moving forward, like a series of checkpoints on your fitness journey.

In this chapter, we've laid the foundation for your goal-setting process. By setting SMART goals, distinguishing between long-term and short-term objectives, and breaking down your aspirations into manageable milestones, you're equipped with the tools to not only dream big but to transform those dreams into attainable, life-changing realities. In the chapters that follow, we'll delve deeper into crafting your fitness plan, ensuring that your goals are not just aspirations but achievable destinations.

Chapter 3: Crafting Your Fitness Plan

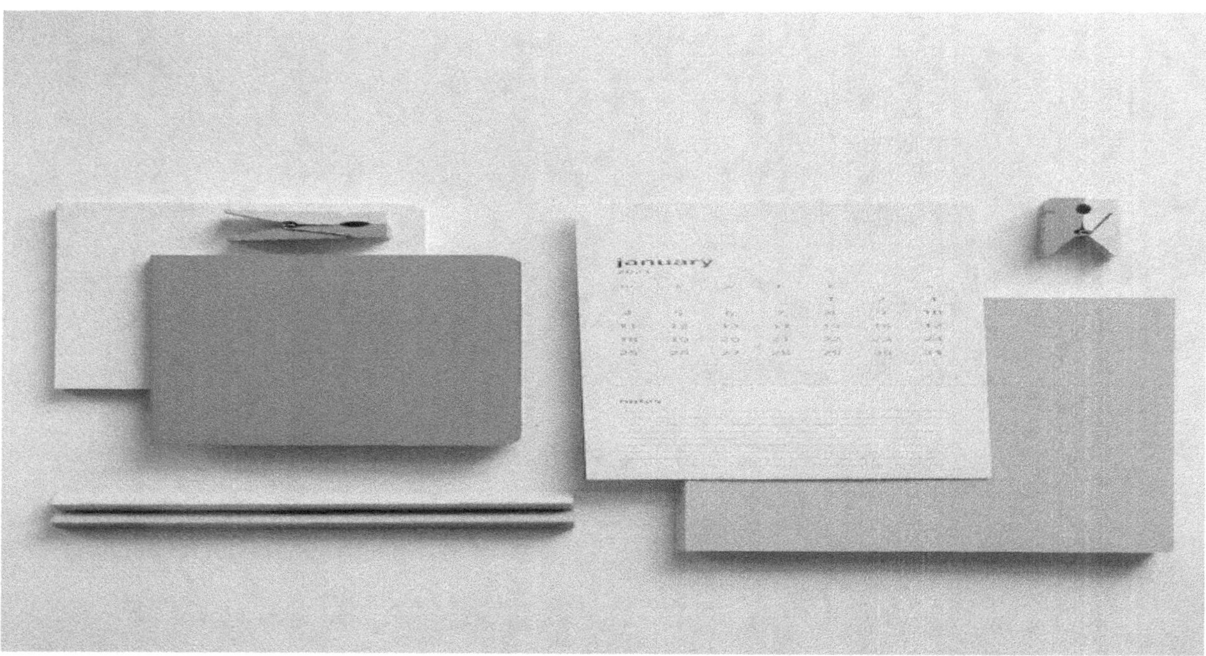

How to Choose the Right Type of Exercise

Fitness is a multifaceted journey, and the path you choose should align with your unique goals and preferences. Before diving into the specifics of crafting your fitness plan, it's crucial to understand how to select the right type of exercise that suits you best.

1. Consider Your Goals: Your choice of exercise should directly align with your fitness goals. If you aim to build strength and muscle, resistance training like weightlifting may be your focus. If fat loss and cardiovascular health are your primary goals, aerobic exercises like running or cycling might be more suitable.

2. Explore Your Interests: Engaging in activities you genuinely enjoy can boost motivation. If you love dancing, consider Zumba or hip-hop classes. If you prefer the outdoors, hiking or swimming might be your calling. Find joy in the journey, and exercise becomes less of a chore and more of a pleasure.

3. Assess Your Physical Abilities: Take into account your current fitness level and any physical limitations you may have. If you're new to exercise or recovering from an injury, low-impact activities like yoga or swimming may be ideal to start with.

Customize a Workout Plan Tailored to Your Goals

Once you've identified the type of exercise that resonates with you, it's time to craft a workout plan that is tailor-made for your goals. One size does not fit all in fitness, so personalize your routine to maximize results and satisfaction.

1. Define Your Frequency: Decide how often you'll work out each week. Consistency is key, so choose a schedule that you can realistically maintain.

2. Determine Duration: The duration of your workouts should align with your goals. For example, longer cardio sessions may be necessary for weight loss, while shorter, intense workouts can be effective for building strength.

3. Select Exercises: Choose specific exercises that target the muscle groups or fitness components you want to improve. For instance, if you're focused on upper body strength, include exercises like push-ups, bench presses, or pull-ups.

4. Set Intensity: Adjust the intensity of your workouts based on your fitness level. Gradually increase the challenge to avoid stagnation. You can do this by adjusting weights, resistance, or speed.

5. Incorporate Progression: Regularly update your workout plan to prevent plateaus. This could involve increasing weights, trying new exercises, or altering workout formats.

Maintain Variety to Prevent Boredom and Plateaus

One of the most common roadblocks on the fitness journey is boredom and plateaus. As your body adapts to a routine, it becomes less responsive to the same exercises. To keep your workouts engaging and your progress steady, embrace variety.

1. Rotate Exercises: Swap out exercises every few weeks to keep your muscles challenged and your workouts exciting. For example, if you've been doing standard squats, try variations like Bulgarian split squats or goblet squats.

2. Change Workout Modalities: Incorporate different workout modalities, such as strength training, cardio, flexibility, and balance exercises. This not only prevents monotony but also ensures comprehensive fitness.

3. Explore New Activities: Periodically explore new activities or classes to rejuvenate your enthusiasm. Trying something novel, like kickboxing, Pilates, or rock climbing, can reignite your passion for fitness.

4. Challenge Your Mind: Incorporate mental challenges into your workouts. For example, try learning a new dance routine, practicing yoga poses, or mastering a new sports skill. Engaging your mind can enhance motivation.

In crafting your fitness plan, remember that it's not just about reaching your destination; it's also about enjoying the journey. By choosing the right type of exercise, customizing your workout plan to your goals, and maintaining variety in your routines, you're creating a roadmap that ensures every step brings you closer to your fitness aspirations. In the chapters ahead, we'll delve into the vital role of nutrition and provide guidance on how to fuel your body for success on your fitness journey.

Chapter 4: Nutrition and Diet for Success

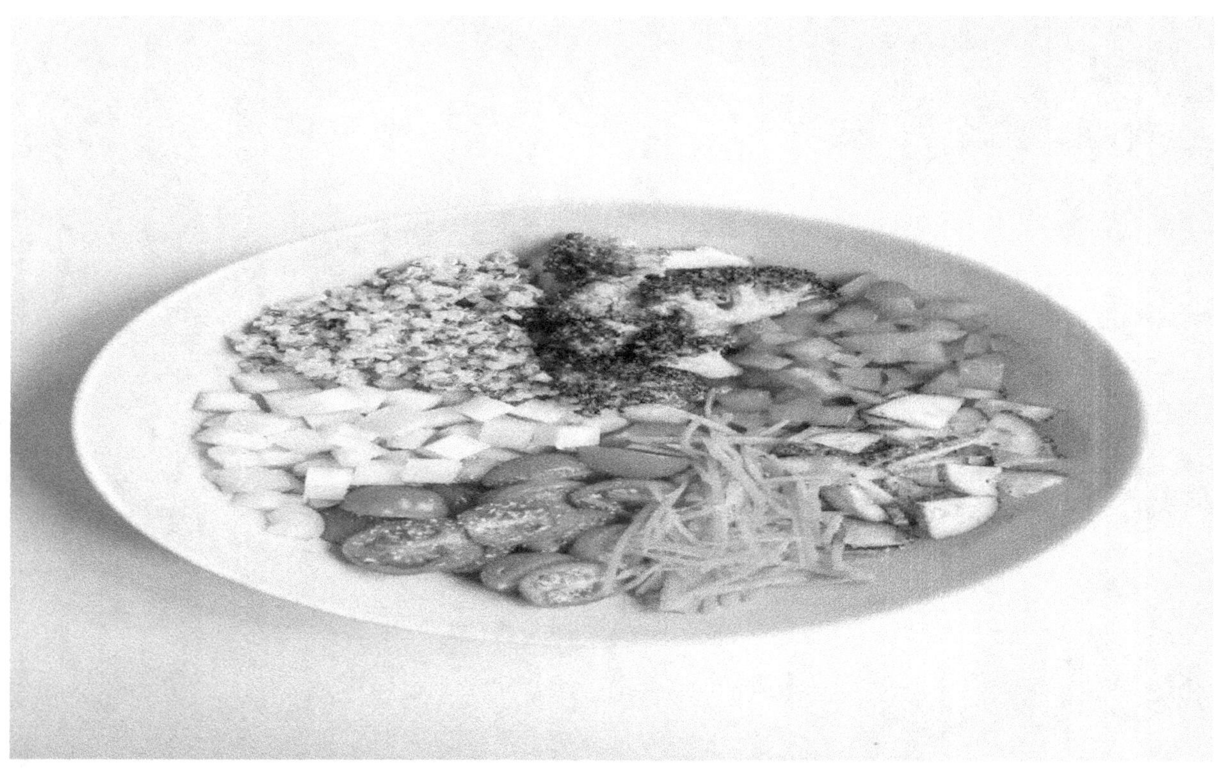

Nutrition: The Foundation of Your Fitness Journey

Imagine your body as a finely tuned machine, and nutrition as the fuel that powers it. Nutrition plays a pivotal role in your fitness journey, influencing not only your physical performance but also your overall well-being. In this chapter, we will explore the significance of nutrition in achieving your fitness goals, the development of healthy eating habits, and effective strategies for planning and tracking your food intake.

The Role of Nutrition in Achieving Your Goals

Your fitness goals are not solely determined by the hours you spend in the gym or on the track; they are profoundly influenced by what you eat.

Nutrition is the cornerstone upon which your fitness success is built. Here's why it matters:

1. Fuel for Your Workouts: The food you consume provides the energy necessary for your workouts. Whether it's cardio, strength training, or flexibility exercises, your body requires the right nutrients to perform at its best.

2. Recovery and Repair: After exercise, your muscles need to repair and grow stronger. Proper nutrition ensures that your body has the building blocks, like protein and essential nutrients, to recover effectively.

3. Weight Management: Nutrition plays a pivotal role in weight loss, maintenance, or muscle gain. The number of calories you consume versus the calories you burn is central to your body composition goals.

4. Overall Health: Good nutrition supports not only your fitness aspirations but also your long-term health. A balanced diet can reduce the risk of chronic diseases, boost immunity, and enhance your quality of life.

Develop Healthy Eating Habits

Achieving your fitness goals isn't about extreme diets or temporary restrictions. It's about cultivating sustainable, healthy eating habits that nourish your body and support your long-term success.

1. Balanced Diet: Aim for a balanced diet that includes a variety of foods from different food groups. Incorporate fruits, vegetables, lean proteins, whole grains, and healthy fats into your meals.

2. Portion Control: Be mindful of portion sizes. Even healthy foods can lead to weight gain if consumed in excess. Use smaller plates, read labels, and pay attention to serving sizes.

3. Meal Timing: Consider your meal timing in relation to your workouts. Eating a balanced meal or snack 1-2 hours before exercise can provide the energy you need, and consuming protein and carbohydrates within 30 minutes after a workout can support recovery.

4. Hydration: Proper hydration is essential for optimal performance and recovery. Drink water throughout the day, and adjust your intake based on activity level and climate.

How to Plan and Track Your Food Intake Effectively

Planning and tracking your food intake is a powerful tool for achieving your fitness goals. It provides awareness and accountability, ensuring that your nutrition aligns with your objectives.

1. Meal Planning: Create a meal plan that aligns with your calorie and nutrient needs. Include a variety of foods to meet your dietary requirements and personal preferences.

2. Food Journaling: Keep a food journal to track what you eat, when you eat it, and portion sizes. This practice enhances self-awareness and helps you identify patterns and areas for improvement.

3. Use Technology: Utilize apps and websites that offer nutrition tracking tools. These can simplify the process by calculating calories and macronutrients for you.

4. Consult a Professional: If you have specific dietary needs or health concerns, consider consulting a registered dietitian or nutritionist. They can provide personalized guidance tailored to your goals.

In this chapter, we've explored the fundamental role of nutrition in your fitness journey, the importance of developing healthy eating habits, and effective strategies for planning and tracking your food intake. Your nutrition choices are the building blocks of your fitness success, and by making informed, sustainable choices, you'll not only achieve your goals but also cultivate a lifelong commitment to health and well-being. In the chapters ahead, we'll address the obstacles that may arise on your fitness journey and provide strategies for overcoming them, ensuring you stay on the path to success.

Chapter 5: Overcoming Obstacles

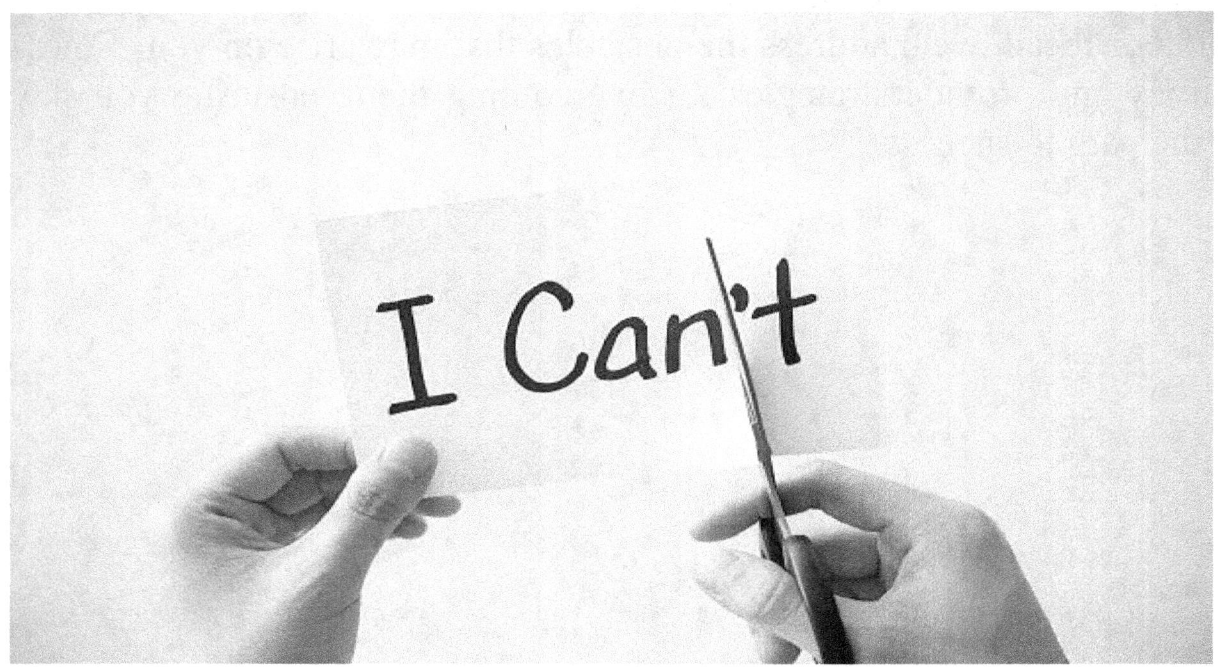

Navigate Common Challenges on Your Journey

Embarking on a fitness journey is an exhilarating adventure, but it's not without its share of challenges. Life is a dynamic journey, and your path to fitness will encounter its fair share of ups and downs. In this chapter, we'll explore common obstacles that often arise and equip you with strategies to navigate them, develop resilience, and overcome setbacks and doubts.

Develop Strategies to Overcome Setbacks and Doubts

1. Plateaus: At some point, you may hit a plateau where your progress seems to stall. Don't be disheartened; plateaus are a natural part of the journey. To overcome them, adjust your workout routine by increasing intensity, trying new exercises, or changing your workout schedule. Refine your nutrition plan, ensuring it aligns with your goals. Seek inspiration from others who have overcome plateaus and remind yourself of how far you've already come.

2. Injury or Illness: Dealing with an injury or illness can be demoralizing. The key is to focus on recovery and adaptability. Consult a healthcare professional for guidance on rehabilitation. Modify your exercise routine to accommodate your condition, and use this time to work on other aspects of your fitness, such as flexibility or mental resilience.

3. Lack of Motivation: There will be days when motivation wanes. It's normal. On such days, lean on discipline and habit. Stick to your workout schedule even if you don't feel like it; once you start, motivation often follows. Surround yourself with motivating influences, whether it's a workout buddy, inspirational quotes, or a playlist of energizing music.

4. Self-Doubt: Doubts can creep in, making you question your abilities and commitment. Combat self-doubt by revisiting your "why" – the reasons you embarked on this journey in the first place. Reflect on past achievements and remind yourself of the progress you've made. Seek support and encouragement from friends, family, or a fitness community.

Build the Resilience Needed to Persevere

1. Mental Toughness: Resilience is not the absence of adversity but the ability to bounce back from it. Cultivate mental toughness by practicing positive self-talk and visualization. Visualize your success, believe in your capabilities, and remind yourself of your past accomplishments.

2. Learn from Setbacks: Every setback is an opportunity for growth. Rather than viewing setbacks as failures, see them as valuable lessons. Analyze what went wrong, adjust your approach, and move forward with newfound knowledge and determination.

3. Seek Support: You don't have to go through this journey alone. Seek support from friends, family, or a fitness community. Surround yourself with individuals who understand your goals and can provide encouragement during challenging times.

4. Stay Flexible: Adaptability is a key component of resilience. Be open to adjusting your goals or strategies as circumstances change. Life is unpredictable, and the ability to pivot and stay committed to your fitness journey will serve you well in the long run.

In overcoming obstacles, you're not only building physical strength but also mental fortitude. Your ability to navigate challenges, develop strategies to overcome setbacks and doubts, and cultivate resilience is a testament to your commitment to achieving your fitness goals. Remember, it's not about whether obstacles arise but how you respond to them that truly defines your success. In the following chapters, we'll explore techniques to stay motivated and maintain your progress, ensuring you stay on course toward your fitness aspirations.

Chapter 6: Staying Motivated

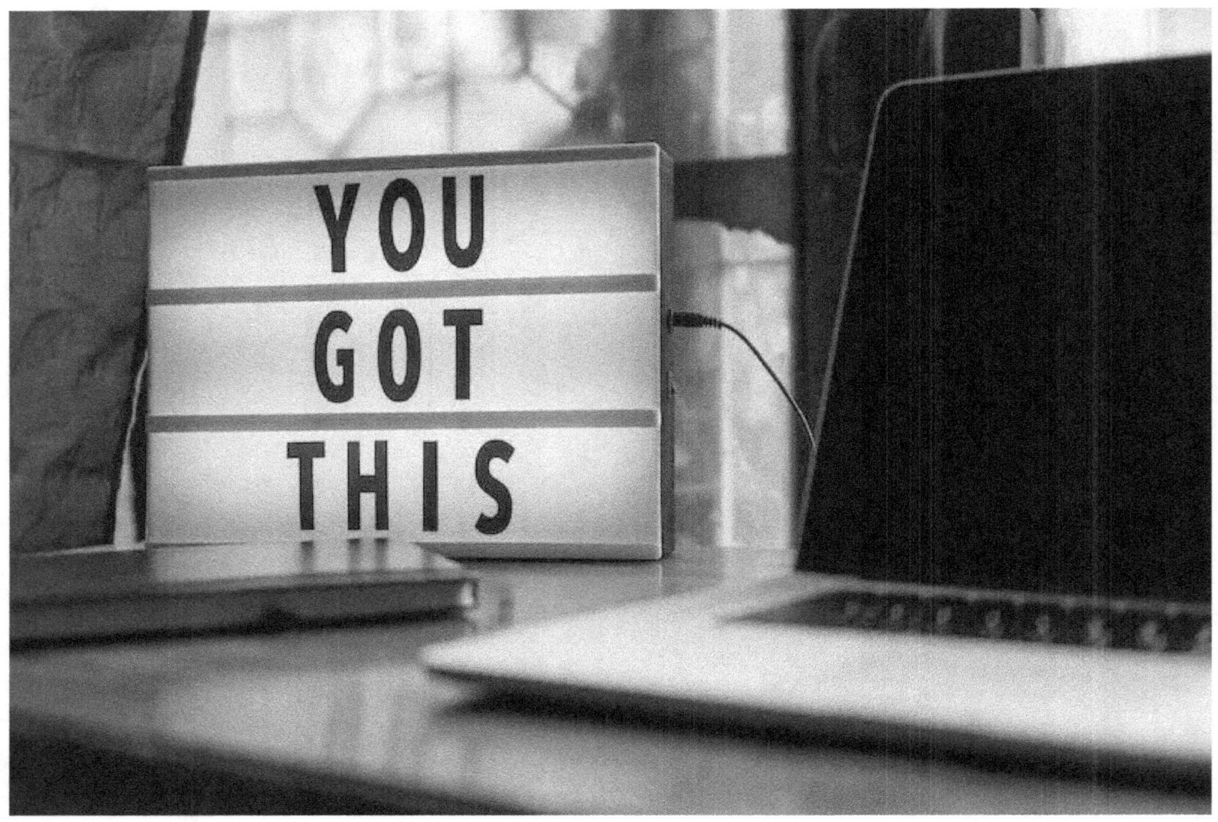

Dive into Motivational Techniques

Motivation is the wind in your fitness sails, propelling you toward your goals. But like the wind, motivation can be fickle, and there will be days when it wanes. In this chapter, we'll explore a variety of motivational techniques to keep your enthusiasm burning brightly throughout your fitness journey.

1. Set Milestones: Break your long-term goals into smaller, achievable milestones. Celebrate each milestone as a marker of your progress. These mini-victories provide a continuous source of motivation and keep you focused on the bigger picture.

2. Visualize Success: Visualization is a powerful tool. Close your eyes and vividly imagine yourself achieving your fitness goals. Feel the satisfaction, joy, and pride as if it has already happened. This mental imagery can boost confidence and motivation.

3. Positive Self-Talk: Monitor your inner dialogue. Replace self-doubt and negativity with positive affirmations. Remind yourself of your strengths and past successes. Use phrases like "I can do this" and "I am making progress" to fuel your motivation.

4. Find Inspiration: Seek inspiration from books, documentaries, or podcasts about fitness journeys and successes. Hearing about others who have overcome similar challenges can reignite your motivation and provide fresh perspectives.

The Power of Visualization

Visualization is a potent technique that taps into the mind's ability to influence our actions. By mentally rehearsing success, you can boost motivation and performance.

1. Create a Mental Movie: Imagine your ideal fitness scenario, whether it's completing a marathon, lifting a certain weight, or achieving a specific body composition. Create a mental movie in which you are the star, and visualize every detail, from the sights and sounds to the emotions you'll experience.

2. Set Specific Goals: Visualization is most effective when linked to specific goals. Clearly define what you want to visualize, whether it's a perfect squat form, a yoga pose, or a successful 10k run.

3. Practice Regularly: Dedicate a few minutes each day to visualization. Find a quiet, distraction-free space and immerse yourself in your mental movie. The more vivid and detailed your visualization, the more powerful its impact.

The Importance of Accountability and Support Systems

Even the most self-motivated individuals benefit from external support systems. Accountability and support are crucial to maintaining motivation.

1. Accountability Partners: Partner with a friend, family member, or colleague who shares your fitness goals. Having someone to report progress to and exercise with can provide an extra layer of motivation and commitment.

2. Online Communities: Join online fitness forums, social media groups, or apps where you can connect with like-minded individuals. Sharing your journey, challenges, and successes with a supportive community can boost motivation and offer valuable insights.

3. Professional Guidance: Consider hiring a personal trainer, coach, or nutritionist. Professionals provide expert guidance, tailored plans, and accountability, ensuring you stay on track and motivated.

4. Regular Check-Ins: Schedule regular check-ins with your accountability partner or coach. These meetings provide an opportunity to reflect on your progress, set new goals, and receive feedback and encouragement.

By diving into motivational techniques, harnessing the power of visualization, and embracing the importance of accountability and support systems, you're fortifying your motivation arsenal. Remember that motivation, like fitness, is a skill that can be developed and nurtured over time. With these tools at your disposal, you'll be better equipped to stay motivated and continue progressing toward your fitness goals. In the next chapter, we'll explore strategies to maintain momentum and make fitness a lifelong commitment.

Chapter 7: Maintaining Momentum

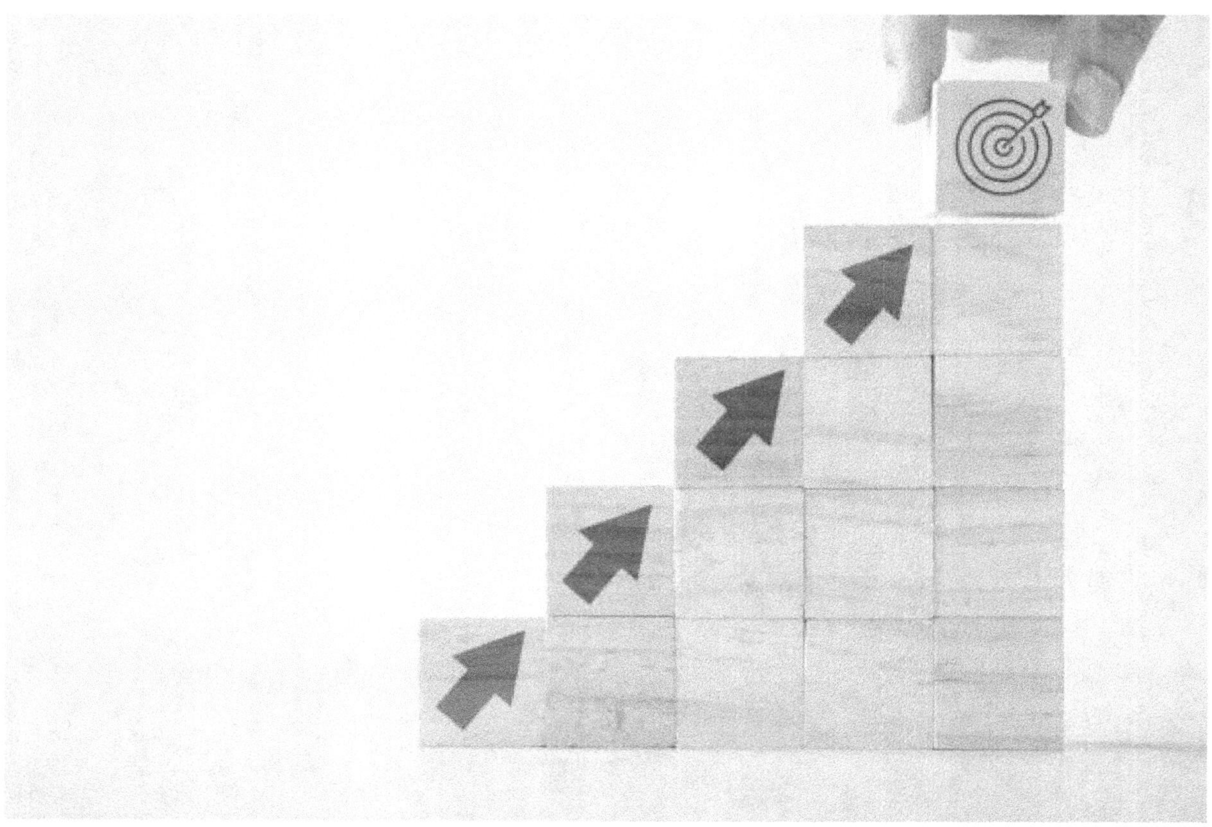

Learn How to Sustain Your Commitment to Fitness

Sustaining your commitment to fitness over the long haul is where the real magic happens. It's about transforming fitness from a goal-oriented pursuit into a lifelong journey that becomes an integral part of who you are. In this chapter, we'll explore how to keep the momentum going, adapt your goals as life evolves, and find the delicate balance that prevents burnout.

1. Embrace the Lifestyle: Shift your perspective from viewing fitness as a means to an end to seeing it as a way of life. Make exercise and healthy eating a part of your daily routine, not just something you do to reach a specific goal.

2. Consistency Over Perfection: Understand that consistency is more important than perfection. There will be days when life gets in the way, and that's okay. What matters most is getting back on track as soon as possible and not letting minor setbacks derail your entire journey.

3. Set New Challenges: As you achieve your initial goals, it's essential to keep the journey exciting by setting new challenges. Whether it's learning a new sport, mastering advanced yoga poses, or competing in a fitness event, constantly challenge yourself to evolve.

Adjust Goals as Life Evolves

Life is a dynamic journey filled with changes and unexpected twists. To maintain momentum, you must be willing to adapt your fitness goals as your circumstances evolve.

1. Life Stages: Recognize that your priorities and available time for fitness may shift as you move through different life stages. What worked in your 20s may not be feasible in your 40s or 50s. Adjust your goals and routines to align with your current reality.

2. Incorporate Variety: Embrace variety in your fitness routine. If you once focused solely on bodybuilding, explore different forms of exercise like swimming, hiking, or dancing. This not only prevents monotony but also accommodates changes in interests and physical capabilities.

3. Set Realistic Expectations: Be realistic about what you can achieve at different stages of life. Your body may not respond the same way it did in your youth, and that's okay. Set goals that challenge you while taking your current circumstances into account.

Find Balance to Avoid Burnout

Fitness should enhance your life, not consume it. Avoiding burnout is essential for maintaining a lifelong commitment to fitness.

1. Rest and Recovery: Prioritize rest and recovery as integral parts of your fitness routine. Overtraining can lead to burnout and injury. Listen to your body and incorporate rest days into your schedule.

2. Quality Over Quantity: It's not about how much you do but how well you do it. Focus on the quality of your workouts and the nourishment you provide your body through nutrition. Quality trumps quantity when it comes to sustaining a healthy lifestyle.

3. Balance Your Life: Fitness is just one facet of your life. Ensure you strike a balance between fitness, work, relationships, and personal time. Neglecting other areas of life in pursuit of fitness can lead to burnout and dissatisfaction.

4. Enjoy the Journey: Remember that fitness is a journey, not a destination. Enjoy the process, relish in the small victories, and appreciate how far you've come. Celebrate your progress, no matter how incremental it may seem.

Maintaining momentum is about embracing fitness as a lifestyle, adapting your goals as life evolves, and finding the equilibrium that prevents burnout. By making fitness an integral part of your life, setting realistic expectations, and enjoying the journey, you're not only ensuring long-term success but also enhancing your overall quality of life. In the final chapter, we'll explore real-life success stories and provide you with a toolkit of resources to support your continued fitness journey.

Chapter 8: Case Studies and Success Stories

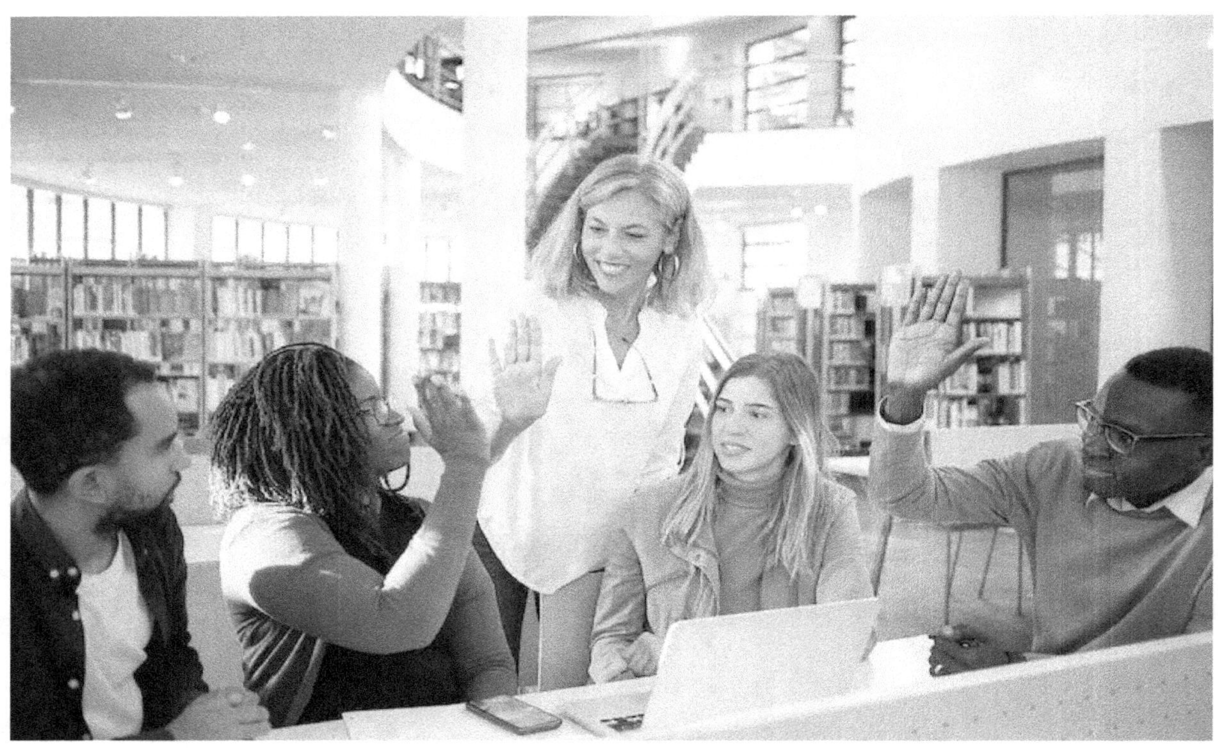

Drawing Inspiration from Real-Life Triumphs

The path to fitness is often paved with determination, commitment, and incredible transformations. In this chapter, we'll delve into inspiring real-life case studies and success stories of individuals who have not only achieved their fitness goals but have also transformed their lives through dedication and perseverance. These stories serve as a source of motivation and offer valuable insights into the strategies that worked for them.

Discovering the Strategies that Worked for Them

Case Study 1: Sarah's Remarkable Transformation

Background: Sarah, a busy mother of two, found herself struggling with weight gain and low energy levels. She felt overwhelmed by her responsibilities and lacked motivation to prioritize her health.

Strategy: Sarah's key to success was integrating fitness into her daily routine. She started with short, at-home workouts during her children's naptime. Over time, she gradually increased the duration and intensity of her workouts. She also focused on meal planning and preparation to ensure she had healthy options readily available. Sarah's dedication to consistency, even during challenging moments, paid off with significant weight loss and increased energy.

Case Study 2: Mark's Marathon Achievement

Background: Mark, a software engineer, set a goal to run a marathon but struggled with staying on track with his training amidst his demanding work schedule.

Strategy: Mark's success story is a testament to prioritizing goals and managing time effectively. He created a detailed training schedule that included early morning runs, lunchtime workouts, and weekend long runs. Mark also joined a local running group to stay motivated and accountable. His gradual progression, commitment to consistency, and support from his running community enabled him to complete his first marathon.

Case Study 3: Emma's Strength Training Triumph

Background: Emma, a retiree in her 60s, wanted to regain strength and independence as she aged.

Strategy: Emma's journey showcases the importance of adapting to individual needs and circumstances. She started with a gentle strength training program designed specifically for seniors. Emma worked closely with a fitness trainer who tailored her workouts to her abilities and goals. Over time, she increased the weight and intensity of her exercises while always prioritizing safety and proper form.

Case Study 4: James' Ongoing Wellness Odyssey

Background: James, a corporate executive, faced the challenge of balancing a demanding job with his fitness aspirations.

Strategy: James's journey underscores the significance of adaptability and resilience. He embraced a flexible workout routine that allowed for both gym sessions and quick home workouts. When work commitments intensified, he adjusted his fitness schedule but never abandoned it entirely. James also sought the support of a nutritionist to optimize his eating habits amidst a hectic lifestyle. His ability to adapt while staying committed to his health goals has resulted in lasting wellness.

These real-life success stories exemplify the diverse paths to fitness achievement. While each individual's journey is unique, they share common threads of dedication, consistency, adaptability, and the pursuit of a healthier, more fulfilling life. By drawing inspiration from these stories and discovering the strategies that worked for them, you'll find valuable insights and motivation to further your own fitness journey. In the final chapter, we'll provide you with a comprehensive toolkit of resources to support your ongoing pursuit of fitness and well-being.

Chapter 9: Resources and Tools

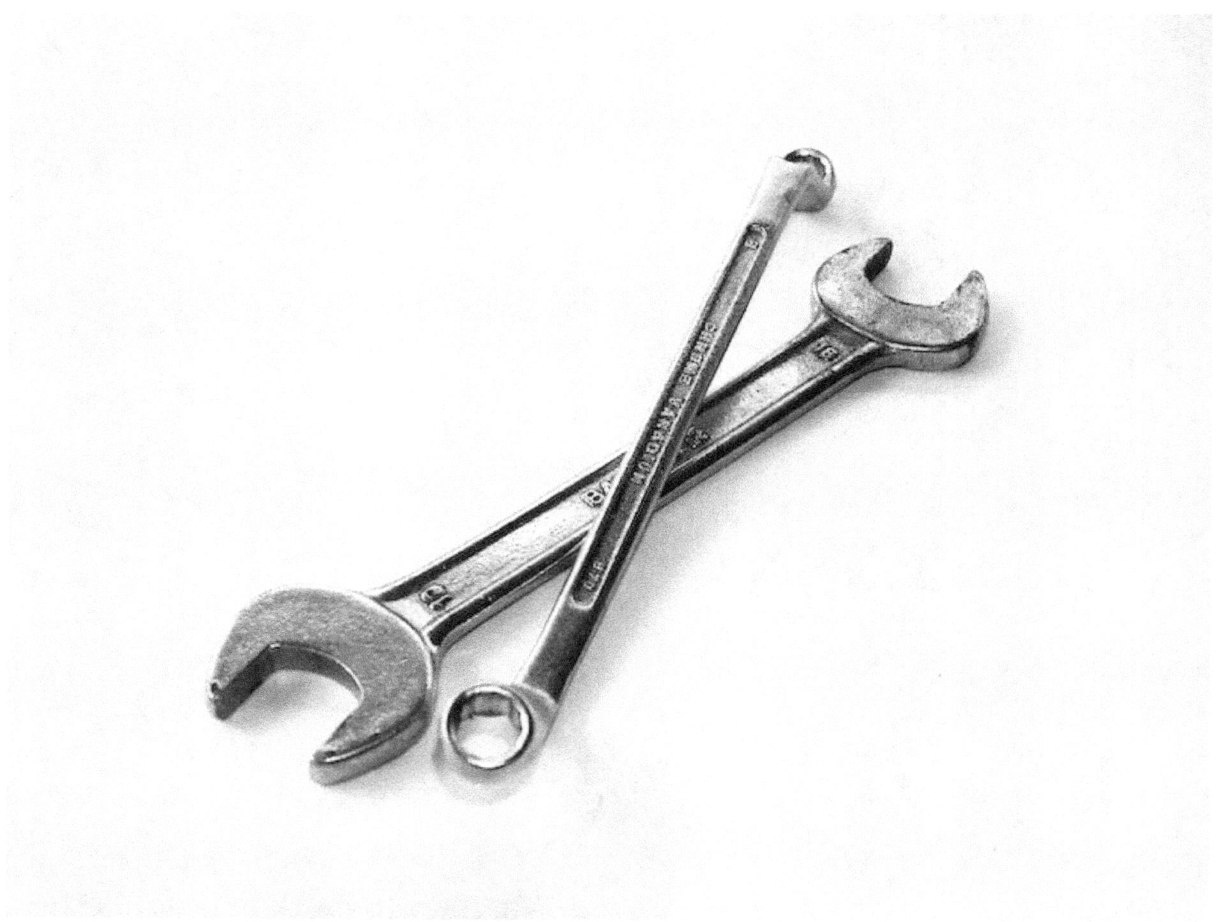

Exploring Your Fitness Toolkit

Embarking on a fitness journey is not a solitary endeavor; it's a process enhanced by the right resources and tools. In this chapter, we'll provide you with a comprehensive fitness toolkit filled with recommended apps, websites, fitness-tracking tools, books, podcasts, and communities that will support and motivate you on your path to success.

Recommended Apps, Websites, and Fitness-Tracking Tools

1. MyFitnessPal: A popular app for tracking nutrition and exercise. It provides a vast database of food items and allows you to set and monitor your calorie and macronutrient goals.

2. Strava: Ideal for runners and cyclists, Strava helps you track your workouts, set goals, and join challenges. It also offers a social component where you can connect with fellow fitness enthusiasts.

3. Fitbit: A versatile wearable device that tracks your steps, heart rate, sleep patterns, and more. The accompanying app provides detailed insights into your activity and health metrics.

4. Nike Training Club: A free app that offers a wide range of guided workouts, from strength training to yoga. It allows you to customize your fitness plan and track your progress.

5. MapMyRun: An app designed for runners and walkers, offering GPS tracking, route planning, and community features. It's excellent for setting and achieving running goals.

Books and Podcasts

1. Book: "Atomic Habits" by James Clear: This book delves into the science of habit formation and offers actionable strategies to build positive fitness habits.

2. Book: "The Power of Now" by Eckhart Tolle: While not a fitness book per se, it explores the importance of being present and can enhance your mental approach to fitness.

3. Podcast: "The School of Greatness" by Lewis Howes: This podcast features inspiring guests from various fields, including fitness and wellness, sharing their insights and journeys to success.

4. Podcast: "The Tony Robbins Podcast" by Tony Robbins: Tony Robbins delves into personal development and motivation, which can be applied to your fitness goals.

Online Communities for Motivation

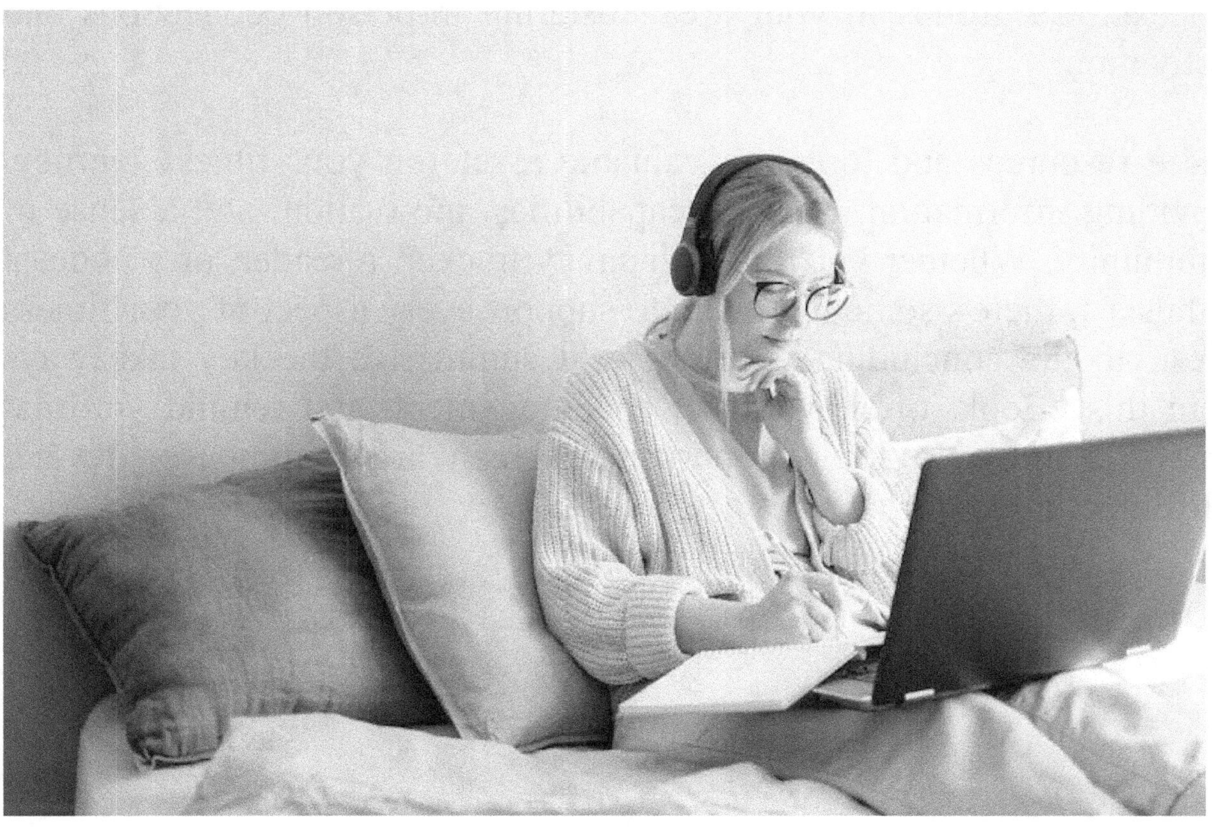

1. Reddit's Fitness Community (r/Fitness): A vibrant online forum where members discuss workouts, nutrition, and share their progress. It's an excellent place to seek advice and motivation.

2. MyFitnessPal Community: A supportive community within the MyFitnessPal app and website where users share their fitness journeys, recipes, and tips.

3. Strava Clubs: Within the Strava app, you can join various clubs based on your interests, from local running groups to virtual cycling communities.

4. Facebook Groups: There are numerous fitness-related Facebook groups catering to different interests and goals. Search for groups aligned with your fitness pursuits.

5. Meetup.com: This platform allows you to find and join local fitness and exercise groups in your area, fostering in-person connections and motivation.

These resources and tools are valuable assets on your fitness journey, providing information, tracking capabilities, motivation, and a sense of community. Whether you're a tech-savvy tracker, a reader, or a podcast enthusiast, there's something here to support every aspect of your fitness quest. In the concluding chapter, we'll summarize the key takeaways from this eBook, offer words of encouragement, and remind you that fitness is indeed a lifelong pursuit that can bring immense joy and fulfillment to your life.

Conclusion: Your Lifelong Fitness Journey

Congratulations on reaching the end of "Fitness Motivation and Goal Setting." Throughout this eBook, we've explored the essential elements that can help you ignite and sustain your motivation, set effective fitness goals, and embark on a lifelong journey toward improved health and well-being. As we conclude this journey together, let's reflect on the key takeaways and offer words of encouragement to inspire your ongoing pursuit of fitness.

Key Takeaways:

1. Discover Your "Why": Understanding your intrinsic motivations, values, and personal reasons for pursuing fitness is the foundation of a successful journey.

2. Set SMART Goals: Transform your aspirations into actionable, specific, measurable, achievable, relevant, and time-bound goals. These clear objectives will guide your efforts effectively.

3. Craft Your Fitness Plan: Choose exercise routines that align with your goals, customize your workout plan, and maintain variety to keep things exciting.

4. Nutrition Matters: Recognize the pivotal role of nutrition in achieving your fitness goals. Develop healthy eating habits, plan your meals, and track your food intake.

5. Overcome Obstacles: Anticipate and navigate common challenges on your journey. Develop strategies to overcome setbacks and doubts while building the resilience needed to persevere.

6. Stay Motivated: Dive into motivational techniques, leverage the power of visualization, and seek accountability and support systems to keep your enthusiasm burning brightly.

7. Maintain Momentum: Transform fitness into a lifelong commitment by embracing it as a lifestyle, adjusting goals as life evolves, and finding balance to prevent burnout.

8. Learn from Success Stories: Draw inspiration from real-life examples of individuals who achieved their fitness goals and discover the strategies that worked for them.

9. Utilize Resources and Tools: Explore recommended apps, websites, fitness-tracking tools, books, podcasts, and online communities to enhance your fitness journey.

Words of Encouragement:

Your fitness journey is not a sprint; it's a lifelong marathon. It's filled with ups, downs, and everything in between. There will be moments of triumph and moments when you question your progress. Remember that setbacks are a natural part of any journey, and they offer opportunities for growth.

Embrace the journey as much as the destination. Relish in the small victories, savor the moments of progress, and keep your "why" at the forefront of your mind. Your motivation may ebb and flow, but your commitment to a healthier, stronger, and more vibrant you is unwavering.

You have the tools, knowledge, and determination to succeed. The path to fitness is not always easy, but it is always worth it. The journey will transform you in ways you can't yet imagine, and it will impact every aspect of your life positively.

So, take the first step or continue the path you've already begun. Whether you're just starting or have been on this journey for years, know that your pursuit of fitness is a lifelong endeavor, and every step you take brings you closer to the best version of yourself.

Thank you for embarking on this journey with "Fitness Motivation and Goal Setting." May your fitness aspirations be realized, your goals exceeded, and your health and well-being elevated to new heights. Your body and mind are capable of incredible feats, and your fitness journey is a testament to your strength, resilience, and determination. Keep moving forward, and embrace the incredible future that awaits you on this lifelong fitness adventure.

About the Author

Eric Uroh is a passionate advocate for health and well-being. With a deep concern for the overall wellness of individuals, Eric has dedicated his life to helping others achieve their health goals and lead happier, more fulfilling lives.

As a fervent fitness enthusiast, Eric Uroh brings a wealth of personal experience and knowledge to the realm of weight loss and healthy living. They have spent countless hours researching, experimenting with various strategies, and engaging in physical activities to discover what truly works for achieving and maintaining a healthy weight. This firsthand experience has given Eric Uroh unique insights into the challenges and triumphs that individuals face on their weight loss journeys.

Eric's unwavering commitment to health and well-being shines through in their writing, coaching, and advocacy work. They believe that everyone has the potential to transform their lives through informed choices and dedicated effort. Through this book, Eric shares his expertise, offering readers a practical and comprehensive guide to achieving their weight loss goals and embracing a healthier and happier lifestyle.

Join Eric Uroh on this transformative journey toward better health and discover the strategies and inspiration you need to embark on your own path to success. Your goals are within reach, and Eric is here to guide you every step of the way.

Books By This Author

Title: Weight Loss Strategies

Unlock the Secrets to Sustainable Weight Loss and a Healthier You!

Are you tired of fad diets and quick fixes that don't deliver lasting results? Are you looking for a comprehensive guide to achieving your weight loss goals while improving your overall well-being? Look no further! "Weight Loss Strategies" is your ultimate resource for embarking on a transformative journey to a healthier and happier life.

Inside this eBook, you'll discover a wealth of knowledge and practical strategies that will empower you to take control of your weight and achieve sustainable results. Say goodbye to the cycle of yo-yo dieting and hello to a balanced, healthier lifestyle.

Here's what you can expect to find within these pages:

- The Science Behind Weight Loss: Understand the fundamentals of weight loss, from caloric deficits to metabolism and body composition. Gain the knowledge you need to make informed choices.

- Nutrition and Diet: Learn the art of healthy eating with insights into balanced diets, portion control, and mindful eating. Explore effective dietary plans, including low-carb diets, the Mediterranean diet, and intermittent fasting.

- Exercise and Physical Activity: Discover the importance of exercise in weight loss and explore various types of physical activities, from cardiovascular workouts to strength training and flexibility exercises. Create a personalized workout plan and learn how to stay consistent with your exercise routines.

- Lifestyle and Behavior Modification: Cultivate healthy habits for weight loss success, including the importance of sleep, stress management, and hydration. Break bad habits such as smoking and excessive alcohol consumption, and build a supportive environment with the help of family and friends or accountability partners.

- Monitoring and Tracking Progress: Unlock the power of progress tracking with insights into why it's crucial to monitor your weight and measurements. Keep a food journal, utilize technology and apps, and adjust your strategies based on your results.

- Dealing with Plateaus and Setbacks: Overcome common hurdles like weight loss plateaus with effective strategies. Learn how to handle setbacks and relapses while maintaining unwavering motivation during challenging times.

- Weight Maintenance: Successfully transition from weight loss to maintenance, develop a sustainable lifestyle, prevent weight regain, and celebrate your achievements and milestones.

In "Weight Loss Strategies," you'll find evidence-based guidance, practical tips, and expert advice to help you navigate the complexities of weight loss. Whether you're a beginner just starting your journey or someone looking to refine their approach, this eBook is your comprehensive roadmap to a healthier, happier life.

Don't wait any longer to take control of your weight and well-being. Get started on your path to success with "Weight Loss Strategies" today! Your transformation begins here.